10 Weight Loss Secrets

for

Busy People

Weight Loss Advice to Take Off Pounds

When Pressed for Time

Ron Kness

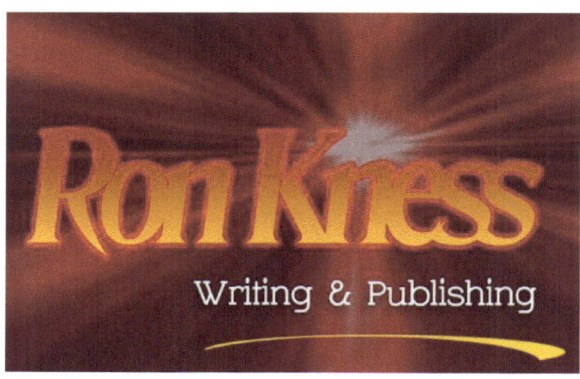

Published by:

Ron Kness

San Tan Valley, AZ

United States of America

ISBN: 9781093607048

Disclaimer

This publication is for informational purposes only and is not intended as medical advice. Medical advice should always be obtained from a qualified medical professional for any health conditions or symptoms associated with them.

Every possible effort has been made in preparing and researching this material. We make no warranties with respect to the accuracy, applicability of its contents or any omissions.

See your healthcare professional before starting any diet, health or exercise program!

Contents

Introduction

Weight loss products, weight loss schemes, weight loss fads can be found everywhere. What is it about weight loss? Why do people want to lose weight? For the millennial who wishes for a 28-hour day, the busy mom who balances between her career and household chores and the deadline-stricken dad, why does weight loss matter?

There are a number of reasons why weight loss is becoming a top in the to-do list of people nowadays. First of all, with all the cancer diagnoses and diseases that are seemingly coming out of nowhere, what people want now is to be healthy. They want bodies that can withstand all the adventures, workload and travels that they plan to enjoy. Second, treatment for any disease is costly. Third, people want to look good and there is nothing wrong with setting lofty personal goals.

Is thin simply in? What is the borderline between healthy thin and unhealthy thin? If you've been doing all suggested schemes to lose weight, then why aren't you losing that excess weight? Moreover, if you have already achieved your ideal weight, what can you do to prevent bouncing back to being overweight?

All these and more are what you are to expect in this book. You will not find weight loss fads here that promise overnight shedding of pounds (you will eventually learn why). This book is more of a journey wherein you get to know yourself and body, find out the right reasons for losing weight and learn to appreciate and love the shape of you in a healthy perspective.

"Only you, your mindset, your discipline, your attitude...can change your BODY."

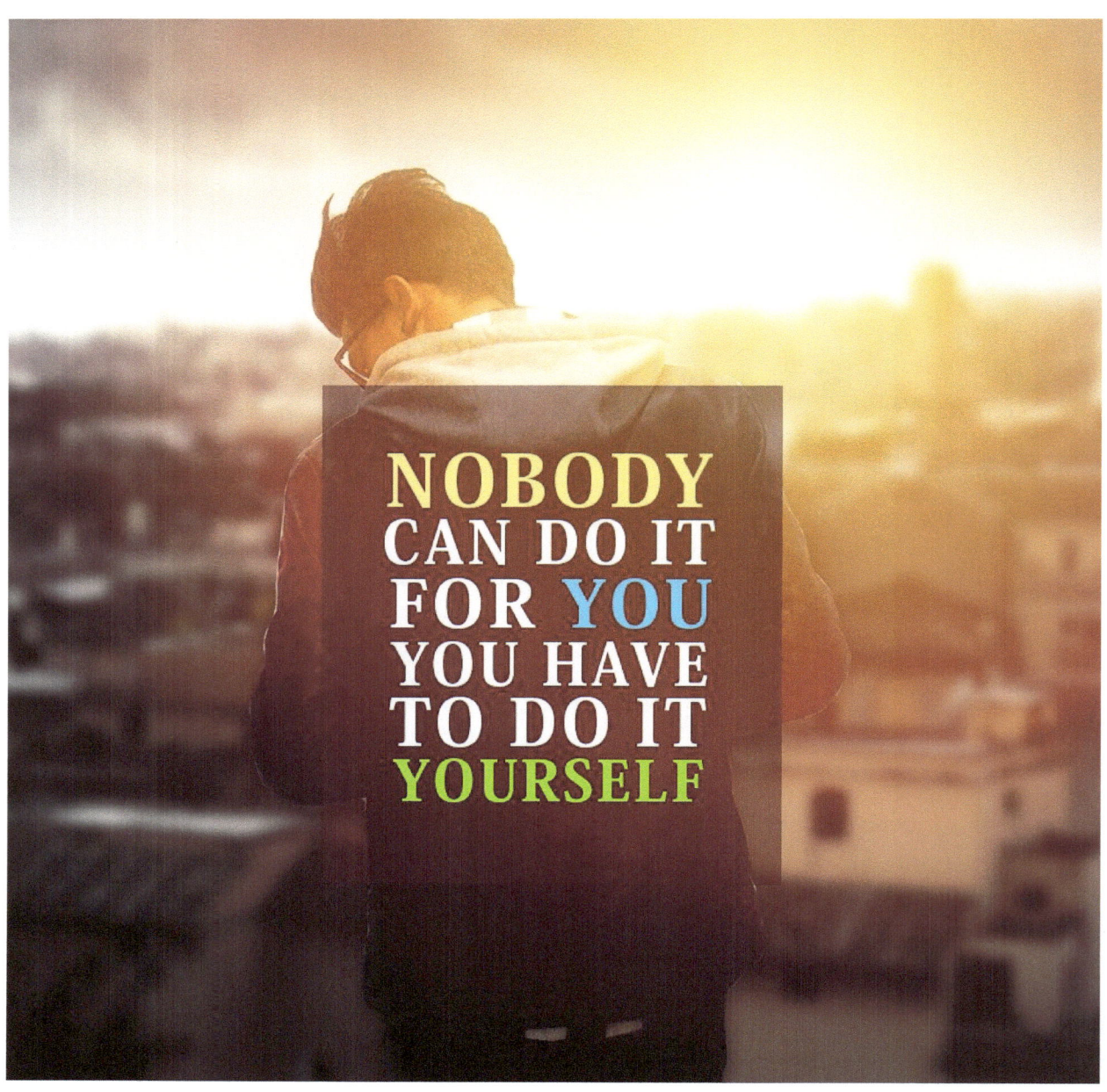

Chapter 1: Why Lose Weight in the First Place

Just type "weight loss" in Google and you will be shown a hundred links to weight loss articles, fads, drinks, potions, shakes, algae and exercise routines that promise a thin you in a matter of days. Desperate people who are really tired of their cellulite may succumb to these suggestions. Though some Google finds are really effective and weight loss may really happen, many will still find themselves bouncing back to their former weight and ending up frustrated. But why is such a scenario a common thing?

The hard truth is losing weight is not easy; especially when you are over the age of 35, dreads workouts, or simply a human who loves food. It is not also a surprise to find teenagers having issues with food and their weight. What I am trying to say here is that, though there are really difficulties that you will encounter in trying to lose weight, the right reasons will lead you the way. What does this mean?

If you are trying to lose weight just because everyone around you looks thin, then you are losing weight for the wrong reason. If, you are trying to shed off pounds just because somebody called you "fat," then you are losing weight for the wrong reason. If, again, you are trying to lose weight just to try something you saw trending on Facebook, then you are doing it for the wrong reason.

Losing weight is a result of your relationship with your body. It is not just meant to be something that will stay with you for a number of days. Losing weight is a lifestyle change and journey that is meant to stay if you are motivated do it for the right reasons.

Here are top reasons why you should consider weight loss for the right reasons:

For health reasons. Obesity is also the root of a number of deadly diseases like diabetes, heart diseases, and kidney problems. To lose weight because you want to be healthy is for the right reason. Being overweight alone is the fifth cause of death worldwide, according to WHO (World Health Organization).

To feel good about yourself. When you feel confident about your body, your perspective and daily mood also follows. You then, will start greeting your mornings with delight and good mood. When you feel light and at ease with the way you are able to move, your day also brightens. And you are able to look in the mirror and appreciate your physical gifts instead of just wishing you look like this or that. Be reminded also, that the link between obesity and depression is medically recognized.

Being overweight means that you are prone to sluggishness and fatigue which are two known factors that contribute to depression. To lose weight because you want to be more thankful for your body and be able to maximize its capacities is one right reason.

To look good. This third reason needs to be understood well. When we say "look good," it does not mean to learn to hide flaws and appear well on the outside. The definition of "looking good" in this perspective means that you are confident with the differences that you have with regards to your body and that of others. It may also mean that you are accepting of your flaws and that you do not dwell on them but instead, you focus on what is beautiful in you.

Another thing, to look good doesn't mean covering yourself with layers of makeup, pads that promises butt enhancements or corsets that make your waist look slim just for the sake of other people's appreciation. To lose weight to be able to fit in clothes that you like and help you move with ease is another right reason to lose weight.

To be fit and improve athletic performance. To become fit may mean that you will be able to participate in more activities that may make you happier. When sweat is released from the body, so are happy hormones. Being able to participate in activities as simple as jogging, for example, is not only good for weight loss but to one's overall well-being to include mental well-being.

The same is true when you are able to trek mountains, bike with friends, swim with your family. Your social life becomes more connected. You are able to enjoy these activities even if you are not the athletic type of person, just some bonding with people in your life who matters. We can really see that indeed, there is a connection between losing weight for the right reasons and being happy.

To improve your quality of life. It is a fact that obesity lessens your quality of life. As mentioned above, your activities and social life can be limited due to the limitations of your body. There are a lot of repercussions that come with these in areas like your social life, self-esteem and may even love life. Let it be clear though, that being fit doesn't necessarily mean you automatically will have an exciting love life.

The point of the matter is that, being fit means that you care for your body and that you feel confident about yourself, this kind of attitude will almost always attract the kind of love that you deserve and not just settle to who's available.

Why lose weight in the first place? Before following any weight loss scheme or before amending your diet, give this time. Reflect first on your reason to make sure that there will be no fall back and that your efforts won't go down the drain. One more important thing to consider is that, the more you know about your body, your limitations and your strengths, the more you are able to choose a weight loss plan that is effective and just right for you.

Notice I didn't say "diet", but a weight loss plan. The difference? A diet is a short-term eating plan where once you come off, the weight you lost comes back on (and usually more), because you are no longer eating food on your diet and reverted back to your former way of eating. If you want to lose a few pounds for a specific function, like a wedding or class reunion, but do not plan on changing your eating habits over the long-term, then a temporary "diet" might be a good choice. Remember, weight loss has to be for the right reason, and if this is *your* reason for wanting to lose (and not to please someone else, then it may be a good choice.

However, a weight-loss plan is a healthy lifestyle change where this is the way you will eat for the rest of your life.

Start with the right reasons and let it be for the right reasons. Let it be for yourself and not for anyone else. Remember that when you choose to do things, be it losing weight or learning something new, when you do it for yourself, the rewards can be more lasting.

This is because you jumped off with the right reasons.

Do not let yourself be pressured with social media and how they picture perfect bodies. You have a unique physique and you have unique gifts. Learn to work with what you have. Accept reality for what is and what is not. Results may take longer than any fad diet, but it surely will not just allow you to lose weight but lose baggage about your body that no longer serve you.

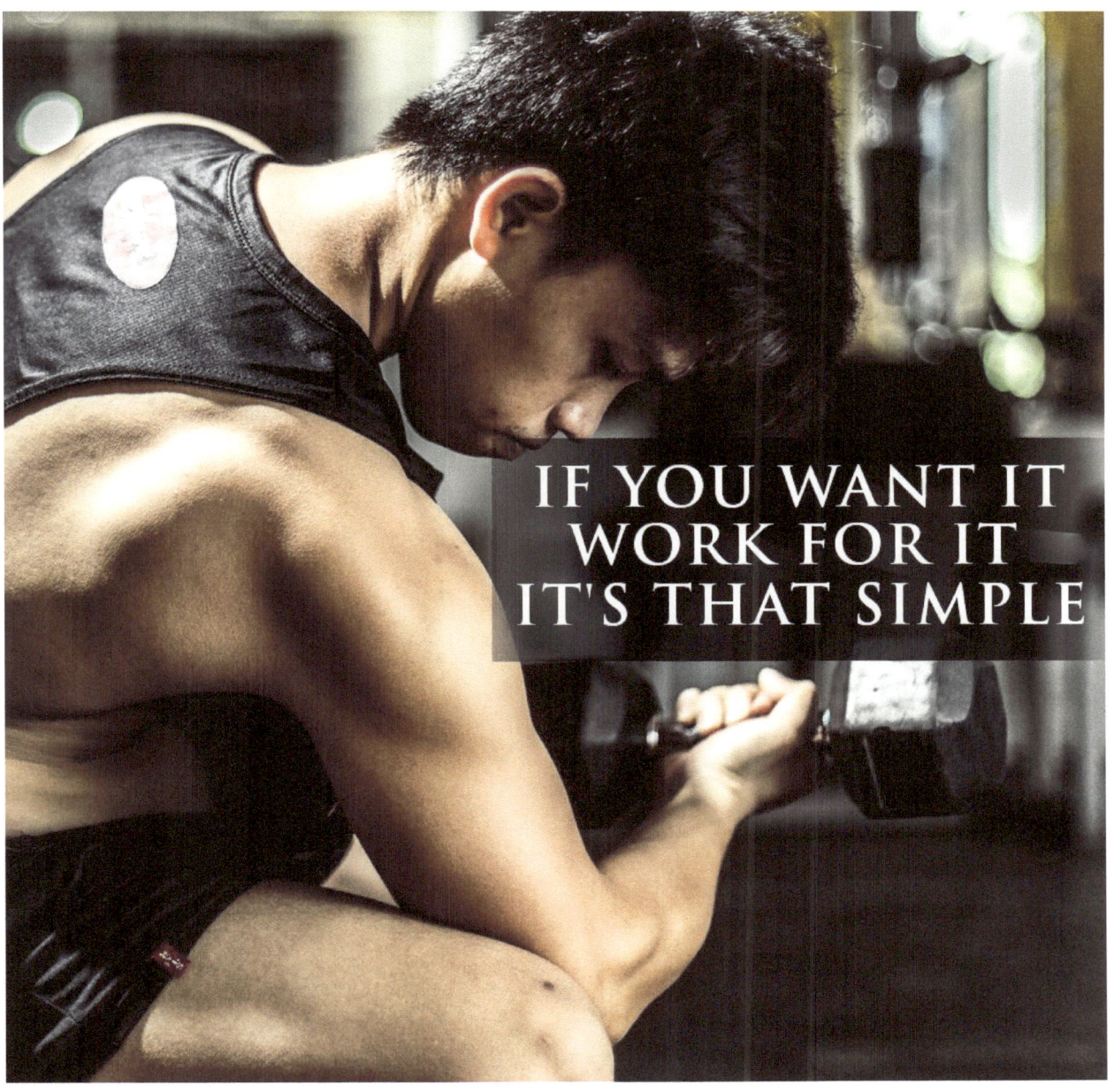

Chapter 2: Why Are You Not Losing Weight

So, if you are reading this book, what I understand is that you are already aware that you need to lose weight and that is the reason you are still here with me. Well, it can be also that you just want to be healthy and want to learn something new apart from fad diets that are all over the internet. Or maybe, you are one who has tried every suggested weight loss program from Google or from fitness instructors and even meal replacement shakes from networking businesses and still you find yourself unable to lose or keep your weight at an ideal level.

What more if you are a busy person who already has a lot on his plate? Where are you to squeeze in gym routines, jog time or how can you cut down on carbs when stress at work and home are "making" you crave for donuts or beer? Below are some of the most common reasons why weight loss, accordingly, is hard to maintain:

- **You started off with the wrong mindset** – you have a beach outing for the weekend and opted to crash-diet for a week. Yes, you instantly got thin, but after the outing, the pounds returned, nastier than before. The hard truth behind the previous scenario is that when you think that weight loss is simply a "fix" and not a long-term health requirement, the pounds bounces back and forth and you always end up frustrated and heavier than before. This is called yo-yo dieting and it is extremely hard on your body. So before deciding on trying any program, make sure that you have the right mindset.

- **Trying hard to follow restrictive diets that are too much for you** – when trying to lose weight, being realistic is also an important factor to consider. For example, you are used to eating whole pizzas for dinner, then suddenly you decided to follow a strict diet fad and shifted from pizzas to celery sticks, what do you think may happen? First of all, your body is not used to small portions of food intake so it will need time to adjust. Second, you are sure to have cravings because it is how detoxification (from too much salt in the pizza) works.

And your frustration list will get longer as you try your best to follow a restrictive diet without proper preparation and mindset. In the long run, this event in your life, especially when you are the busy type, will contribute more to weight gain instead of it helping you lose weight.

- **Not taking seriously mindful and sustainable habits that is crucial in any weight loss program** - the hard-core truth is, any weight loss program is actually based on the willpower of the person wanting to lose weight. It is not dependent to the kind of program, to a fitness instructor or even a strict diet. This is because no matter how effective a plan may be, if you do not have the will to sustain it, its recommendations and restrictions, it will be all for nothing. No one's gaining anything and efforts will simply go down the drain.

Why aren't you losing weight? To keep yourself from getting frustrated, here are tips you can still try to make you understand weight loss beyond the superficial:

- **Accept that there is no alternative to exercising regularly**: got excited when you saw that massage belt that is supposed to melt your abdominal fats while you watch T.V.? Believe me, I saw that too and thought of getting my credit card quick. What stopped me, then? The human in me wants to believe that massage belts are manna from heaven, but in reality, I know that no massage belt or anything for that matter could literally melt my abdominal fat the way abstaining from carbs and doing push-ups can do. That is another hard-core truth.

  The good news is, there are a lot of types of exercise in this world. All you must do is to find one that suits you. If you love sweat, there's the gym option. If you are one who loves to be alone, you can jog with your IPod. If you are not one who appreciates equipment, then you may opt for Yoga or dancing as weight loss tool. If your busy schedule won't allow classes, then you could opt for YouTube tutorials or sessions via DVD's. The important thing is you find something you like to do and have time to move that body of yours on a regular (and consistent) basis.

- **Before getting frustrated, make sure you have no medical condition that makes you gain weight no matter what you do** – let's take matters intelligently. Before putting the blame on yourself and hating the universe for making you fat, make sure that you do not have underlying medical conditions like hormonal imbalance, hypothyroidism or depression. These conditions will add to your weight no matter how hard you try. So it is best to be medically cleared first before starting on any weight loss plan.

- **Believe that there is a strong connection between sleep and weight gain** – these two are seemingly distant to each other but you are about to learn that they are indeed, best of friends. When you lack sleep, there is a BIG possibility that you are to become overweight. This is again, a hard-core truth and one reason for such is that, when you lack sleep, there is a great chance that your food choices are those that will make you gain weight. And you can attribute that to the fact that lack of sleep affects your ability to make healthy food choices. Another thing to consider is that, lack of sleep also affects your metabolism rate.

- **Make water your best friend** – keeping yourself hydrated helps you lose weight. First, drinking water before a meal gives you the feeling of being full so chances are, you will lose that hefty appetite of yours and eat less. Drinking water also increases your metabolism so there is a greater chance of not gaining weight back that is lost. This being said, it is high time to make sure that you are drinking at least eight 8-ounce cups of water (just a little over 2 liters) daily. Monitor it and be serious about it. Also, another thing to motivate you is the fact that the benefits of drinking water are aplenty, not only in terms of metabolism and weight loss but to your overall health as well.

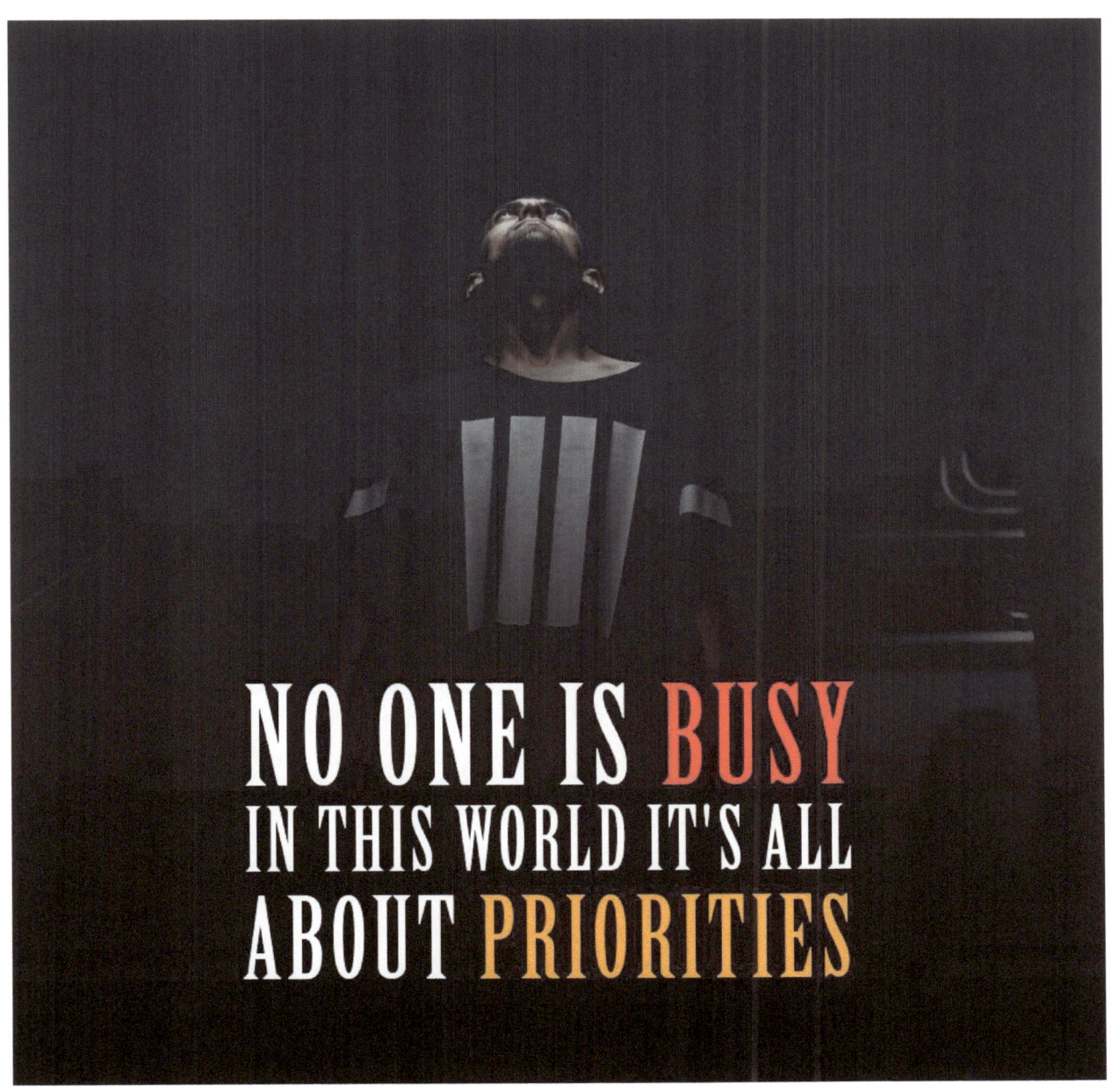

Chapter 3: When Losing Weight Becomes Unhealthy

Losing weight is supposed to be one healthy goal. It is a beautiful yet difficult journey to start with. It begins with the acknowledgment that indeed, your weight needs trimming. Then, you try to find a weight loss program that suits your lifestyle. Next, you are accepting that the journey may take longer than quick fixes but is meant to stay. And then you stick to it until it becomes a habit, a part of your daily routine. This may sound ideal however, it is obviously slower.

Quick fixes with regards to losing weight are abundant in the internet ... but none of them work over the long-term. There are even schemes wherein you are to starve yourself and rely on tablets which are supposed to melt your fat away. Others involve products that may eliminate fat but have a gruesome effect on your body. Here are sample of weight loss fads to avoid:

Diuretics – these are pills that are supposed to flush sodium and water out of one's body. It is intended for other concerns though some are using it for weight loss. This is one dangerous step as it may damage your kidneys and make you dehydrated. Although, yes it may make you lose weight in no time, the weight lost is almost all water weight. In the last chapter we talked about the benefits of staying hydrated. Diuretics do just the opposite – make you dehydrated. Yet people keep buying them. Don't fall for the hype. The damage it can cause is not worth your effort.

Caffeine supplements – companies that make this tablet claim that since caffeine boosts metabolism and has fat-burning magic, this tablet is the answer to your weight loss difficulty. But they seemingly forgot to mention too much caffeine also causes anxiety, sleep problems and rapid heartbeat. Again, in the last chapter we talked about the strong sleep weight loss connection which is counterproductive with these tablets. At the end of the day, relying on these tablets for weight loss is not worth the money and effort.

Waist trimmers – though an instant hit among millennials who want find push-ups a punishment, this corset-like device may look cute but is actually dangerous. Though it is possible that you may achieve an hour-like body sometime in the future, sadly, your internal organs will have to suffer first. Wearing waist trimmers may cause acid reflux, impair breathing, cause heartburn and GI problems. If it really can push fat out your system is yet to be discovered.

Sauna suits – this was designed by companies to lure those who can't stand hard work plus sweat, so they invented this device that is supposed to make you sweat by the ton with minimal effort. The risks include stroke, low blood pressure from overheating, unnecessary pressure to the internal organs and dehydration. This is just to remind us that indeed, there is no shortcut to exercising and sweating.

Tongue patch – believe it or not, some are really that desperate that they are willing to undergo a procedure that involves putting a patch in their tongues to make chewing painful. The goal is to make you want to consume liquids only. This procedure guarantees fast weight loss, but the repercussions include psychological and physiological risks. If weight loss is supposed to be a beautiful journey, then there is actually no need to inflict pain in yourself.

Weight loss tea – this is being advertised as a magic potion that is supposed to eliminate fat. All you have to do is to drink as much as you can. Indeed, it is too good to be true. Like the previously mentioned caffeine tablets, there is harm in succumbing to this because of a lot of reasons. One is that, the safety in the manufacture of this products are quite unsure especially now that "diet teas" gained popularity. The consumption of inorganic teas which are potentially loaded with pesticides and consumed in large amounts can cause harm to one's body. One thing more is the fact that its effect when it comes to weight loss is yet to be proven scientifically.

Okay, I get it. You are busy. You have no time to consult experts nor do hours of researching. So how may you know if you are clicking the bait for a fad weight loss hula boo? Here are easy tips to keep in mind when spotting a fad diet product:

1. Weight loss is based on taking pills, powders, special juices or herbs – You may now be wondering, "what's wrong with all these?" Though they all are seemingly a healthy alternative, after all, herbs, for example has been around for ages. The truth with these fads is that they are just gimmicks that will trim down your wallet and not your belly fat. Some may even post danger to your health especially those that promise instant weight loss.

Pills that are being marketed usually contain laxatives or diuretics that forces your body to eliminate. Though due to frequent visits in the toilet and dehydration, you may really lose weight fast, the effect it will have on your body is simply not worth it.

2. Weight loss is based on drastically cutting back on calories – Again, is this not the way it should be, you may ask. Please read the sentence again and notice the word "drastically." A healthy diet plan should not require or make you starve. Not only will hunger make you a bitter person, believe me, it will also have not-so-good-rebounds. Scientifically, our bodies are not designed to shed off pounds of more than one or two per week. Here's one fact to keep in mind, our bodies react to starvation by means of dumping water out of our system. So, when we starve ourselves, what we are actually losing is water and not fats. Still, it is better to stick to diet plans that are non-instant but are healthy and will surely last. But then they are not diet plans and instead healthy lifestyle choices.

3.Weight loss is based on skipping meals and replacing them with special shakes/drinks or food bars – The problem with this kind of fad is that you are missing out on specific food groups which are vital for your health. This scheme doesn't support healthy weight loss and will have its repercussions later. Keep in mind that what you are aiming for is a healthy body, that is the main reason why you want to lose weight and not deprive yourself and binge-eat after. Another thing to consider is that, there is no scientific proof that such meal replacements are enough to keep your vital organs properly functioning.

4. Weight loss plans that promises instant results – Like that of instant everything, instant weight loss has its fallback. If what you are about to adhere to is too good to be true, then I think it's time to trust your guts and accept that indeed, satisfying results only come from hard work. Think of how long you gained the weight you want to shed, it took a number of months or years right? So, it is just fair not to expect your body to lose in a week what it took months or years to gain.

5. Weigh loss plans that never mentions lifestyle or change in mentality – This is the easiest to spot yet the hardest to recognize. One sure thing that makes a diet plan successful and true to its goal is the mention of a lifestyle change or a shift in mentality. The reason for such is that, fads simply want a sale, an income. Whereas, real weight loss advocates of fitness instructors are aware that without a change in lifestyle, weight loss may turn to be something frustrating, endangering (health wise) and short-term.

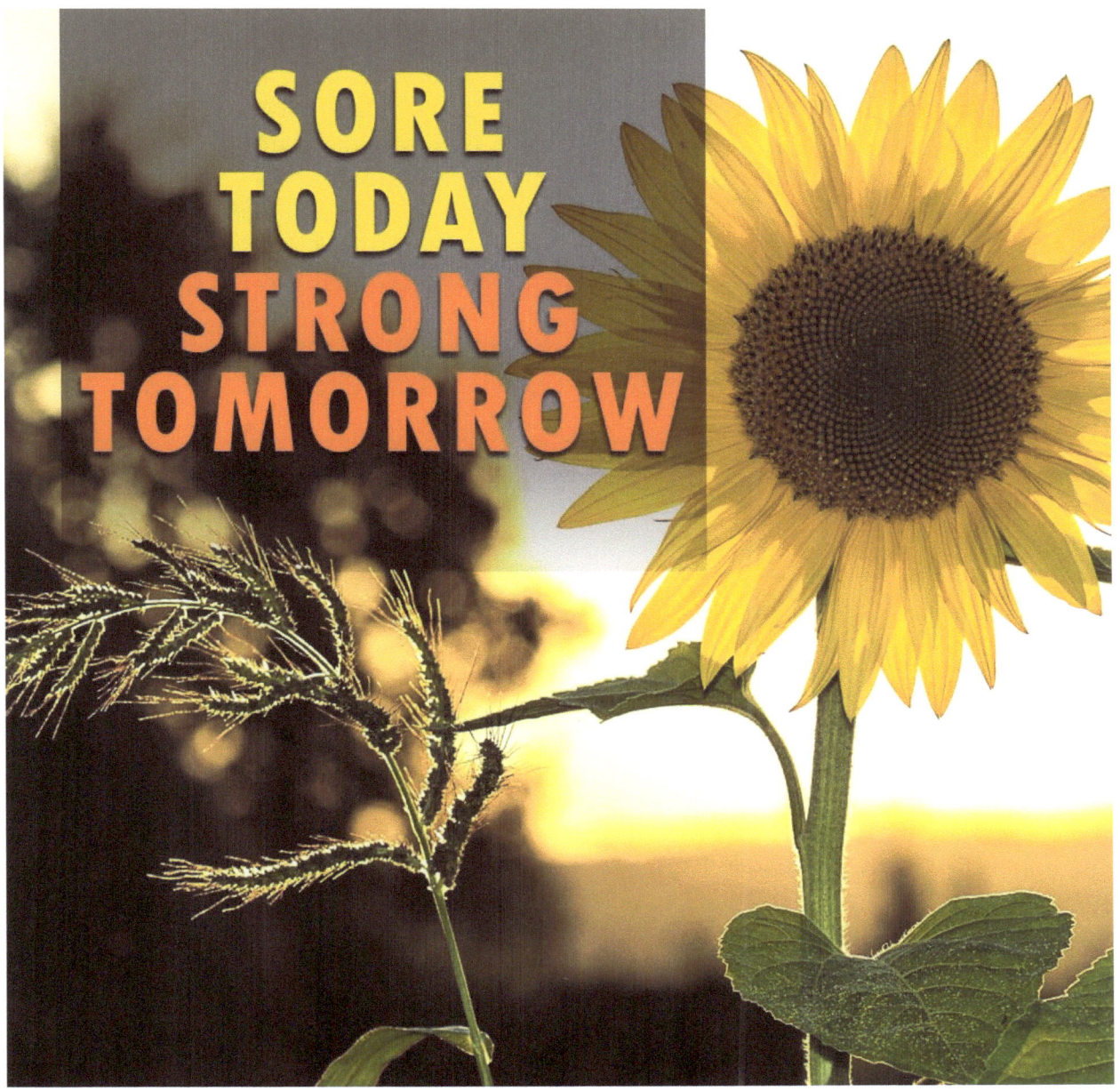

Chapter 4: A Realistic Game Plan

A maximum of two pounds a week is what is considered healthy when it comes to losing weight, according to experts. Keep this in mind if what you are aiming for is a weight loss plan that will not cause you health issues later on. This kind of recommended pacing with regards to losing pounds also is one that most probably will last.

But, do you ever wonder at times, why there are instances where you followed a regimen religiously but still the result you are expecting is far from becoming a reality? Have you experienced feeling like that of a goat after eating all the recommended greens in a particular diet plan and yet, your flabby arms and beer belly still greets you in the morning? Either of these experiences lead to a frustrating ordeal or the tendency to succumb to fad diets that promises instant results. Both of which are unhealthy – physically and mentally.

Now, have you ever wondered why this happens at all? What could be the reason? Have you heard of different body types? Let's discuss this further and find out its connection to losing weight. The truth is, for certain body types, certain food will have certain effects. And yes, this means to say that it is possible for your friend to eat all the ice cream she wants and not gain weight while your other friend, or you, simply cannot.

Another truth to be considered is the connection between your metabolic rate and body type. It is the determining factor of your lean muscle and body fat percentage. It also a way of knowing which food will keep your weight and which won't. Here is a list of the different body types...find out which one is yours!

The Apple Body Type: Do you tend to carry a lot of extra weight around your belly area? Do you notice that although you are gaining weight, your legs/lower body part tend to stay slim? If you have answered yes, then you now know your body type. The challenge with this type of body is that the accumulation of visceral fats in the abdominal area attracts a lot of diseases: diabetes, heart diseases and types of cancers. This accumulation of fat also lowers one's metabolic rate making it hard to lose weight and tends to make the whole body inflamed. For people with this body type, a low glycemic diet is recommended.

Not only will it keep body weight in its track, it will also keep diseases away. Food that's great for this body type are the following:

- legumes

- nuts

- green leafy vegetables

- fruits

- lentils

It is advised to stay away from the following:

- white bread

- donuts

- snacks with artificial sweeteners

- soda

- pastries

- pasta

- cookies

An important tip for people with this body type is "healthy snacking." Not only will this practice prevent sugar spikes, it will prevent unhealthy binges that add up to belly fat.

The Inverted Triangle Shaped Body: People with this type tend to store fats in the upper part of their body. They usually have broad shoulders and slim lower body part. They are sometimes referred to as "top heavy" body type. The key for these people is to choose complex over simple carbs. What does this mean? It is simply choosing quinoa and oats versus white rice and potatoes. Aside from that, choosing leafy greens over cheeses and processed food that are high in sodium are the options that will surely make a person with this body type lose weight. Another thing to remember is to load up on magnesium which can be found abundantly in black beans and spinach. This is to ensure that efforts on weight loss is not thrown in the garbage bin.

The Pencil-Shaped Body: If you are one who have same measurements for your shoulders, waist and hips, and have a hard time looking for curves – you have found your body type name - the pencil-shaped body. This is the skinny type of people who, when they do gain weight, tends to accumulate everything in their belly. Again, like those who have an apple-shaped body, this type of fat accumulation is dangerous to one's health and is a magnet for diseases. Pencil types need to make sure that they are getting three full meals a day. A plate where there is a balance of skinless chicken, for example, brown rice and side greens. Keep in mind that it is possible to be skinny and have a healthy BMI but still have a high percentage of body fat. People with this type of body, since they are prone to being skinny-looking already, needs to focus instead in achieving a toned physique and lowering their body fat percentage.

The Pear-Shaped Body: Literally akin to the shape of the pear fruit, people with this type of body carry most of their weight in the lower portion of their body. The type of fat that this type tends to accumulate is called subcutaneous fat or simply the type of fat that can be pinched. The difference between pear-shaped and apple-shaped bodies is the kind of fat that they tend to have. Though the body fat of Pear-shapes are not as dangerous as apple shapes, their fats tend to be stubborn. It is harder to trim off.

So people of this body type needs more serious weight loss regimens than their counterparts. To help shed off fats in the abdominal region, a high-protein, lean meat diet is recommended. Brown rice and whole wheat bread are helpful. The consumption of the following should be avoided by Pear-shapes: alcohol and other drinks like lattes and fruit shakes that load up calories instead of quenching thirst, food that are high in hormones like chicken wings because this makes losing weight very difficult.

The Hour-Glass Shaped Body: They say that this type of body is the ideal as it tends to have body fats that are evenly distributed. Though, of course, it is also very possible for this body type to gain weight and the areas that usually load up fats are in the face, waist, knees, cheeks and arm area. People of this body type should be reminded that they are prone to inflammation. As such, food that trigger inflammation should be avoided – dairy, processed food, snacks that are rich in sugar and salty food. Like other body types fiber-rich food like green leafy vegetables, whole food (farm to table), and lean meats are advantageous to hour-glass shaped bodies.

The truth of the matter is, we are all born unique and different from each other. But, are connected in one way or another. Confusing as it may sound, it is what it is. What I am trying to say here is that, it is inevitable that we are born with the body types that we have. It is not our choosing.

But, what we can do about it is to focus on our body's strengths and to keep it healthy so that it may be able to serve its purpose the best way it can. As we decide to alter our diet to achieve weight loss, let us not forget the other half of losing weight which is exercise. There is no alternative to moving our physical body.

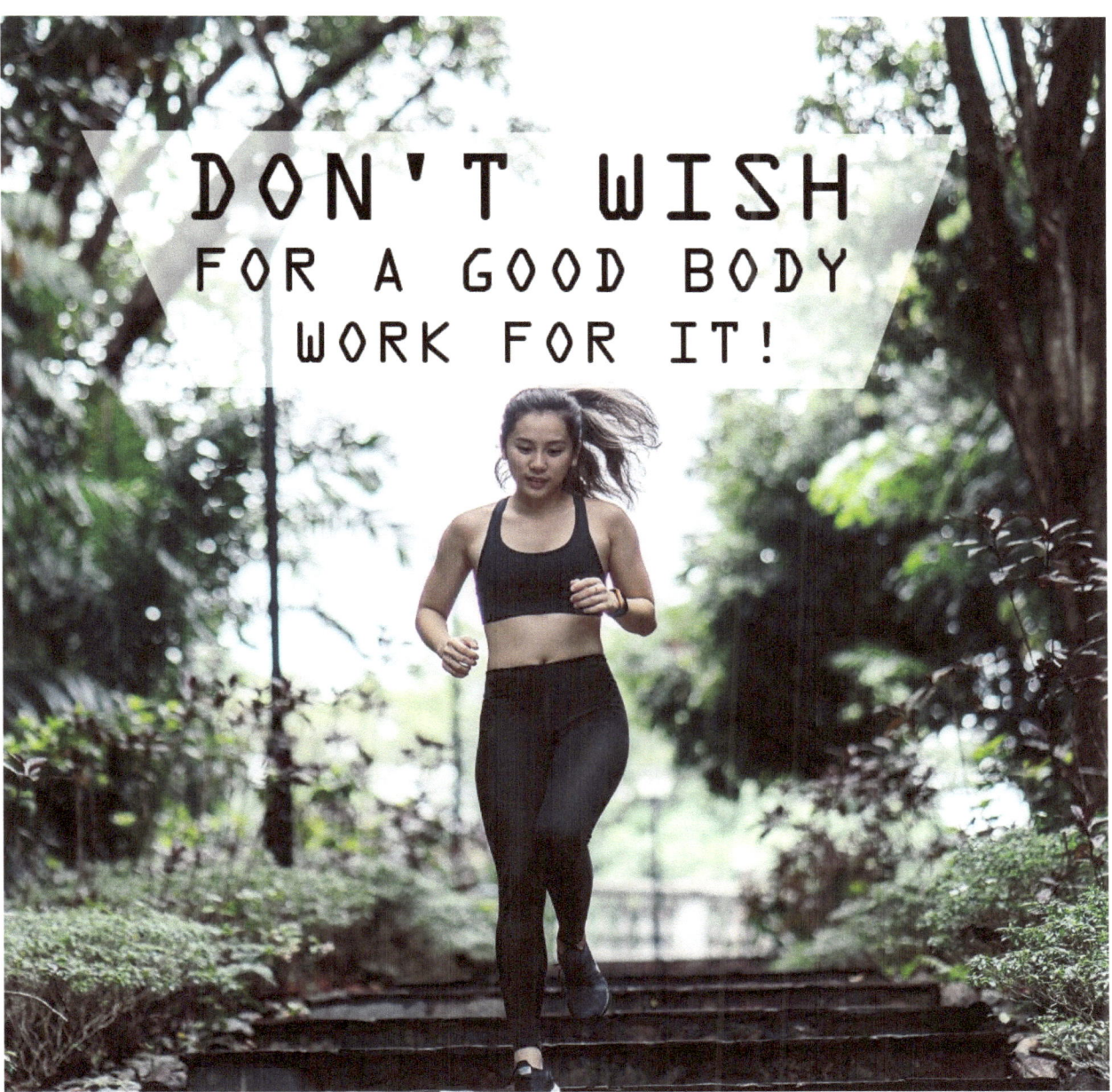

Chapter 5: Hype or Truth: A Closer Look at Popular Health Products

I couldn't blame you if have a stock of tubs of yogurts you bought in the supermarket thinking that is a healthy weight loss alternative to pancakes for your breakfast. If you are the busy type and you have no time to really do researches, and the internet and some health magazines scattered in your office market recommend such products, there is really a great chance that you will believe all the hype. Well, forgive yourself. These ads are designed to do that, and you were caught on the bait.

The fact is, there are a lot of food/products being marketed as healthy alternatives to weight loss but are really just wasting your money and worse, making your belly fat bigger. Remember that salad-go-green hype? Yes, leafy greens are on top when it comes to weight loss but the dressings that come with it should not be included if a flatter belly is what you aim for. Maybe they just forgot to mention that in their popular weight loss blogs. A slip.

Thanks to the internet, connections are much easier. Just one disadvantage though, fake news is also on the rise. And if you are not smart enough recognize what is real and what is not, chances are you will be "hyped." Here is a list of popular products claiming instant weight loss that one should avoid:

Frozen yogurt versus Greek yogurt – What's the deal among all these kinds of yogurt taking the internet by storm? Let make it simple: Greek yogurt is the real thing (unsweetened and sour), frozen yogurt usually found in supermarkets is a lighter version of the ice cream (sweet and creamy). So, if what you are aiming for is weight loss, then better stick with the real thing. This will not only save you money but also will not make you wonder where all those belly fats are coming from.

Vitamin water versus water – These vitamin-infused bottled waters are new in supermarket shelves. But what's the hype about? It is simply water with flavor that is spiked with added nutrients that claim may aid in weight loss. Experts claim that there is actually no need to shell out extra cash for this. The reason?

If you are serious in losing weight, chances are, you have already altered your diet to healthier alternatives, thus, there is no reason to make these infused water bottles part of your daily routine. And that one should be aware of the hidden high sugar content and preservatives mostly found in these bottles.

Quinoa and brown rice versus white rice – When trying to lose weight, we try to avoid carbs and sugar. Opting for quinoa as an addition to salads and snacks and making brown rice a staple in our daily meals is not considered a hype. This is because both alternatives are higher in fiber and protein content and low in sugar than their counterparts, making weight loss more manageable.

Probiotic drinks versus fermented vegetables – The truth is, both are good for the health and yes, there is a possibility that they can aid in weight loss. How so? Gut health is important not only in weight loss but one's overall health. Probiotics and fermented products aid in the promotion of a healthy gut through helping it have a healthier balance between its good and bad bacteria. And when there is good balance in the gut, absorption of nutrients becomes easy for the body. This means less craving for comfort food: deep-fried potato fries, salty chips, vanilla ice cream, donuts, etc.

Granola bars versus good old peanuts – Granola bars are basically a mixture of different kinds of nuts glued with sugar. Good old peanuts are bought either raw or cooked already, can be boiled or fried. Granola bars recently gained its popularity when hikers and other sports enthusiasts started promoting it as a meal replacement when one is in the middle of hike or biking competition. They claim it provides the energy needed for quite a number of hours. This claim didn't slip from ears of those aiming for weight loss. Granola bars became a substitute for snacks and sometimes, even dinners. Though nuts are innately nutritious, what weight watchers should watch when opting for these bars are its sugar, sodium and fat content so as not to defeat the purpose of skipping a meal.

Cow's milk versus almond milk – Aside from the fact that one is vegan and the other is not, again, the factor to consider when trying to lose weight is a product's fat content. Of course, because almond milk is plant-based, more or less, its fat content is lesser than its animal-based counterpart. The question is though, why is there a need for milk in your diet? If you are one who needs it for shakes and breakfast puddings, then the healthier alternative is the almond milk. But if you can survive with just your greens, you are better off. Cow's milk is in hot seat right now as a lot of studies are being made and the results are somewhat disturbing.

There are studies that show how cow's milk is associated with the formation and aggravation of mucus leading to respiratory problems, different kinds of allergies and hormonal imbalances. So, just to be safe when you are trying to lose weight, opt for plant-based milks if there is really a need for milk at all.

Dark chocolate versus milk chocolate – Chocolates have been around for a long time. Some poets even described it as food for the gods. And like other things, living and non-living in this universe, it also evolved. Cacao, where it is derived from, has nothing to offer but nutrients and good stuff to its harvesters. However, man, the curios one, tried adding a bit of this and that to cacao until the name "chocolate" was born. Today, there is what we call dark chocolate (sans milk, nuts, etc.). Nutritionists call it the real chocolate. While there is what we also call, the milk chocolate which, true to its word, has milk, sugar and all other stuff which makes the simple cacao seem unhealthy. Of course, a small amount of milk chocolate won't harm a healthy person, but when one is aiming for weight loss, then the better option is what is termed dark chocolate.

Beer versus red wine – When caught in a social gathering or when you simply want a sip of an alcoholic drink, what is the "healthier" option between the two? The challenge here is the calorie content especially when losing weight is in effect. Beer, especially those that are homegrown (not mass produced) and brewed or crafted in your local towns, are fermented to perfection and have nutrients of its own. Red wine, on the other hand, is also known to do good for those with heart ailments. I think that the point here is for the drinker to be aware of the amount of beer or wine he drinks rather than compare which is the healthier alternative. Another thing to consider that is of importance is the side dish that comes with the drinking. Cheeses and olives are a great addition to calorie counting when partnered with wine or beer.

Red meat versus white meat – Red meat usually comes from beef or pork while white meat usually comes from chicken. But which is healthier when it comes to weight loss? Energy wise, when you are into the athletic side and are burning a lot of calories from all the sweating, red meat gives more energy as compared to white meat. When it comes to weight loss, red meat is loaded with B vitamins and helps a lot in achieving your goal. Though, it comes with a hefty price when compared to white meat. When it comes to muscle building, white meat poses greater chances. This is because white meat is easier to digest making nutrients easier to absorb and muscle-building faster too. So when choosing between the two, think of your goals and budget. Keep in mind that when trying to lose weight, portioning is the key when it comes to all kinds of meat. Just make sure that what you have on your plate is enough to keep you going all day.

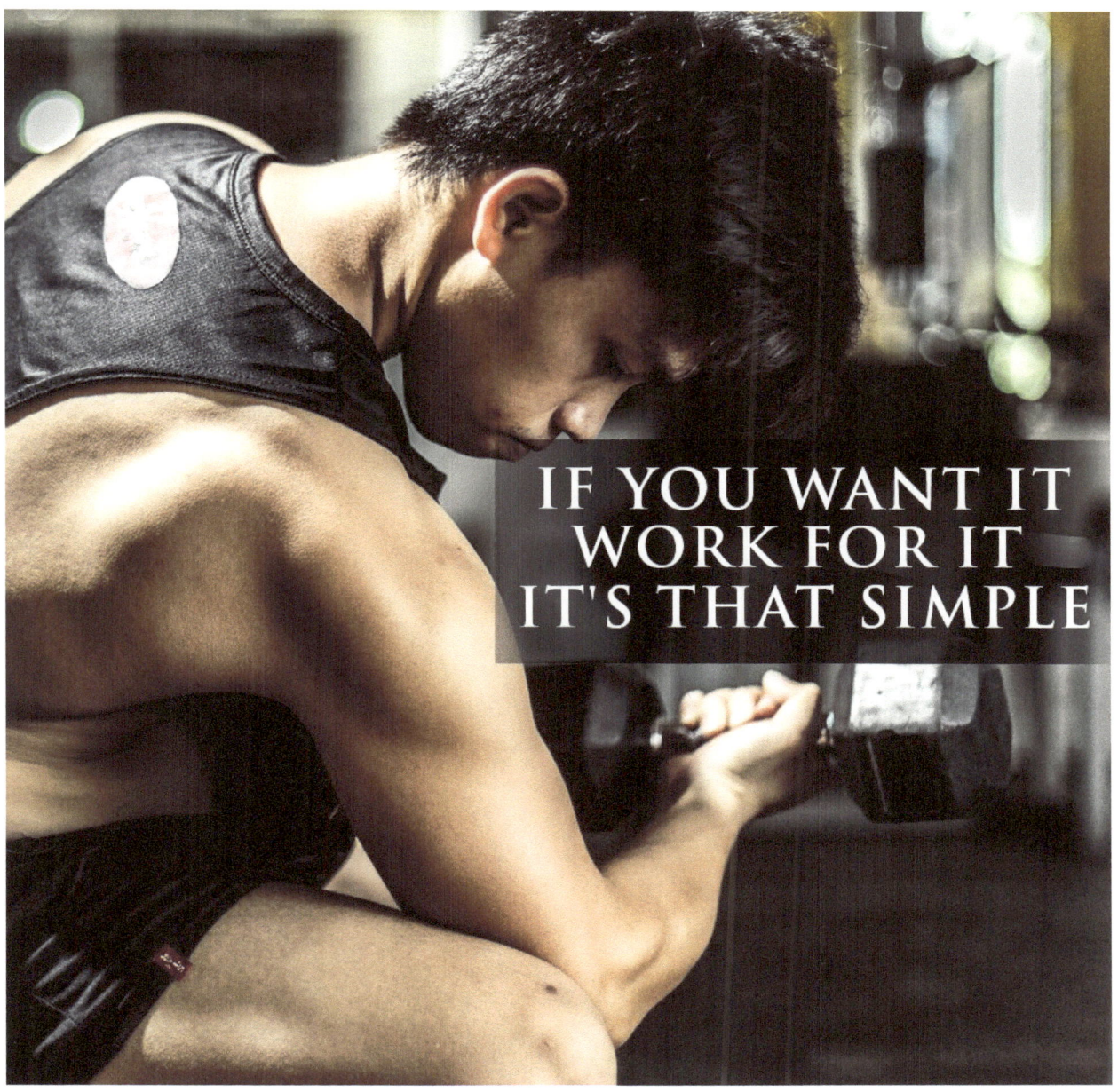

Chapter 6: Shed Fats Slowly But Surely

As mentioned earlier, there are a lot of factors to consider when trying to lose weight. There is the motivational goal, one's body type, learning to spot fad products and a lot more. Now that you are more grounded, I hope, in your plans and goals, it is high time to have a sneak peek at some of the most popular fad diets in the market and internet today. This is to make sure that before you decide on a diet regimen, you are at least closer to what is really effective, tried and tested and not just some gimmick designed to squeeze your hard-earned cash.

It is also a wise move to be reminded there are also diet plans that causes trouble more than eliminate unwanted fats in the body. Here are a few samples of it:

Diet plans that focuses on eating from one food group for a period of time. A classic example would be consuming green smoothies, and only green smoothies for a period of time until you have achieved your ideal weight. Smoothies are supposed to be healthy but if used in the wrong way, it can affect the health in various ways. It is a fact that we all have different body types and therefore, needs according to body type also differs.

 Another fad in the internet is what is termed to as the "Sirtfood Diet." This type of diet encourages the consumption of food rich in polyphenols (kale, buckwheat, red wine, etc.), the goal is to trigger one's metabolism and promises that weight loss is sure to follow. What is bleak in this diet is that, although it can be that weight loss may happen, the longevity of its effect is in question. This is because this diet plan is based on a 3-week time frame and for experts, it may cause nutrient deficiency as the recommended food is not well-rounded. It is still best to look for a diet plan that may be slow to show results but is geared toward a long term effect.

The coconut-oil-everything diet is also taking desperate wannabe-thin-instantly by storm. This type of diet plan encourages the use of coconut oil or the replacement of everything to coconut oil. Although, coconut oil can be healthy, again, if used properly. There is also a concern among experts because coconut oil has a high saturated fat content. The alternatives they recommend are alternating coconut oil with avocado or virgin olive oil.

Fasting versus dieting. Nowadays, these two terms seemingly "married" each other especially to those seeking a fast result with regards to their weight woes. Fasting is defined in a different light when it comes to religious beliefs and practices. Fasting, medically is also seen as a need depending on doctor's recommendation. Diet, on the other hand, is the consumption of food on regular interval with weight loss and sometimes health concern as the main reason. The point of the matter is, if one chooses to use the other i.e. fasting but the end goal is that of dieting. It is when the two are interchanged that chaos may follow.

The raw food diet. This type of diet believes that heat, especially when cooking, destroys essential nutrients in food, hence eating everything raw is the way to go. Though it may sound extreme and might also limit one's food choices, the biggest trouble this imposes, especially to busy people is the amount of time it takes to do. To be able to adhere to a complete raw food diet, a lot of juicing, germinating, hydrating and sprouting needs to be done. With regards to it being effective, yes, one can say that raw food may be more nutritious than its counterparts but cooking food doesn't also mean no nutrients at all. So like with many other things, the key is balance. A good example is to have raw food during day offs and holidays and sticking to cooked food for the rest of the week. This way, weight loss may be more effective and less stressful.

The Master Cleanse of the lemonade diet. This diet plan involves replacing all meals with a mixture of maple syrup, cayenne pepper and lemon juice and water for 10 days. The goal is to cleanse the body from toxins and reset the bodily functions. Although this type of diet has been around for decades, not consulting a health expert before doing it may expose you to a lot of dangers. Those who have already tried this cleanse claim to have experienced hallucinations, severe hunger and dehydration among other stuff. This is also seen as a type of diuretic since you are only to consume liquid. As a result, you will also shed water and once you finish the cleanse and start eating solid food again, there is a greater chance that you will binge-eat and gain weight faster than before.

The Sleeping Beauty diet. You may think that this is something funny, but sad to say, it has taken the internet by storm. Celebrities even promote this extreme form of dieting. The philosophy is that, when you are asleep, then you are not eating and as a result, you are to get thin. As lame as it sounds, many who are desperate to see their pounds shed off have already tried this fad. The practice of this diet involves ingesting sleeping pills that of course, will make you sleep for hours to prevent you from eating anything. The fallback of course, is when you wake up and couldn't control yourself to eat. Chances are, you might eat more than what you usually have.

And a riskier chance is that, overdosing on sleeping pills might make you not wake up at all. Ever.

The tapeworm diet. You read it right. This diet involves a tapeworm. One is to ingest tapeworm eggs and wait until it grows into a real, adult tapeworm and be able to eat all the food being eaten by its host. As absurd and extreme as it may sound, this fad has followers. Medically speaking, it is unhealthy to have a tapeworm inside one's body moreover rely on it for one's weight loss goals. Parasites absorb nutrients and not fats, although it may cause weight loss, but the reason for such is because you are depriving yourself of essential nutrients and feeding it all to a tapeworm inside your body. Keep in mind that there are a lot of healthier alternatives to weight loss that doesn't involve a parasite.

The cookie diet. This may sound enticing to most readers... who wouldn't want to eat cookies and get thin in the process? The fallback is, most probably, the type of cookie that is in your mind is one that is loaded with sugar, chocolate and milk. But in this diet plan, the kind of cookie that you will be chewing on for breakfast, lunch and dinner are the hard, unsweetened, high-fiber, high-protein type. The goal is to control your calorie intake. This type of diet may seem effective at first but, most practitioners find themselves binge-eating at nighttime. Still, it is better to eat real food and just be wary of portioning and calories.

The cabbage soup diet. They say that this is the mother of all fad diets that is circulating all around the internet. This diet plan involves replacing meals with fat-free cabbage soup with bananas or skim milk as snacks. Though many practitioners claim that they, indeed experienced weight loss, the longevity of it is in question. This diet plan works because you are ingesting a low-calorie diet that is full of water and fiber which gives the feeling of fullness. But still, it is considered an instant fix. Aside from that, long term effect of adhering to this diet plan may cause chronic bloating and loss of lean body mass. Hence, a diet plan such as this should still be balanced out with other food like lean protein, healthy fats and carbohydrates.

The HCG diet. This type of diet plan involves taking the HCG (human chorionic gonadotropin). A hormone that is supposed to suppress appetite. This is considered an extreme weight loss scheme as it promotes severe starvation in order to achieve weight loss. The main purpose of injecting this hormone is to treat fertility issues in women. Its role in weight loss is not medically recognized.

The cotton ball diet. A fad diet borne in social media channels, chat rooms and fake news websites. The idea of the initiators is to soak cotton balls bought in supermarkets or anywhere else ordinary cotton balls are available and ingest it. This diet plan is literally asking its followers to eat "flavored" cotton balls. To some it may sound absurd, but a number of people have already tried it and claim that they have indeed experienced weight loss. Though it is possible to actually lose weight, it is no denying that there are also disadvantages. First and foremost, a cotton ball is not under any food group so it is simply not considered food. Second, it is unsafe for human consumption due to the simple reason that commercial cotton balls are not made up of cotton but of synthetic fibers, not to mention that some are even bleached. All these chemicals added to cotton balls poses a lot of dangers to the human body. Medically speaking, replacing regular meals with cotton balls deprives the body from essential nutrients that can only come from real food (fruits whole grains and vegetables). In essence, this fad diet can create chaos inside and outside of one's body. Try your very best to stay away from it.

The Five-bite diet. Another fad, this diet asks you to follow a rule: you may eat everything you want or desire...but you can have just five bites of it. It sounds more psychological than logical. You may not feel deprived as you can eat whatever you want, but it takes a great discipline on your part to make sure that you are to have only five bites. Whether or not this diet is effective, short term or long term, is not yet defined. But, surprisingly, it already has gained quite a number of followers. If you are serious about getting fit and losing weight, this is definitely not worth your time.

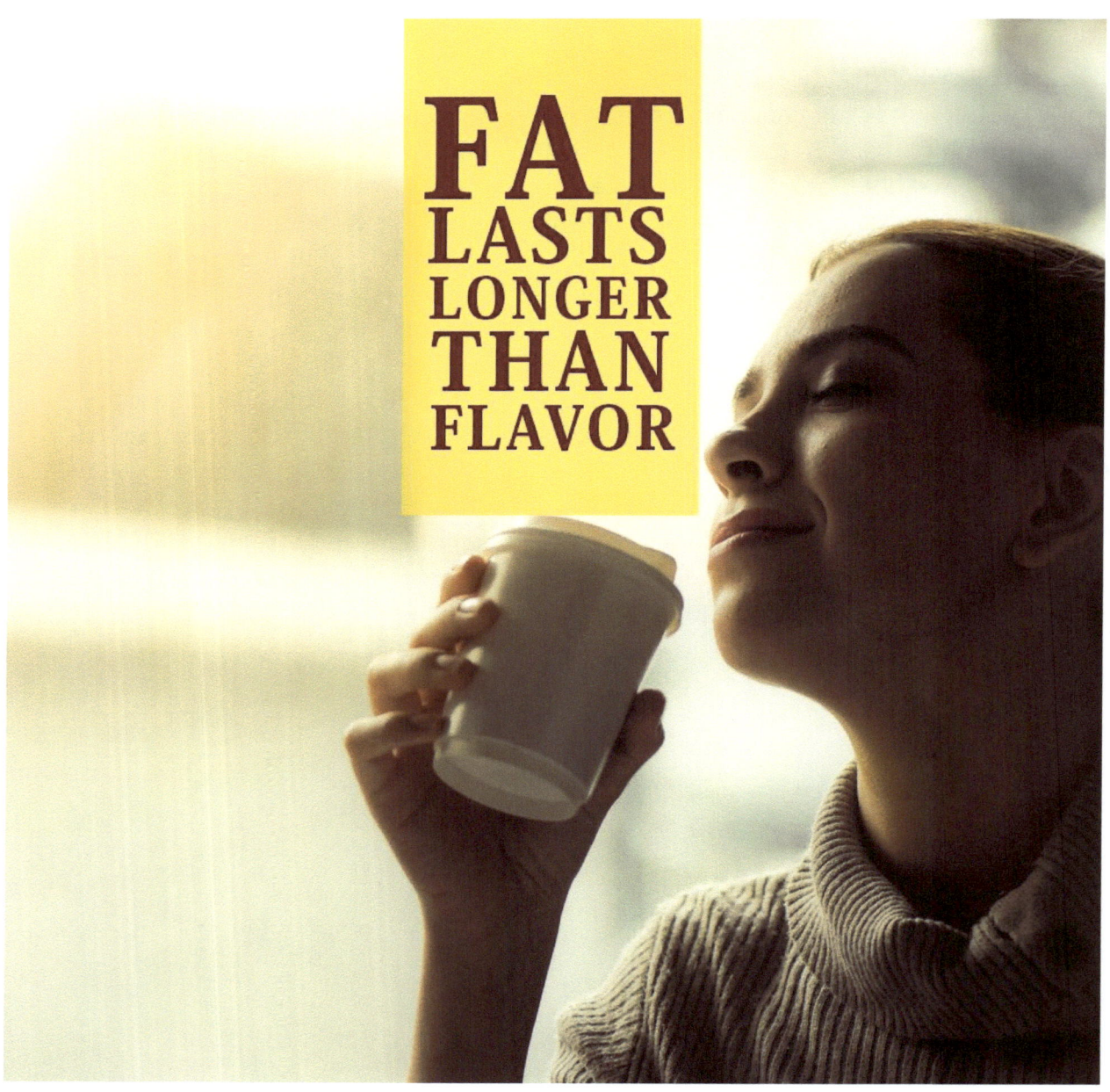

Chapter 7: Intense, Flexible or Cardio Workout: Choose What Suits Your Lifestyle

Whether you're a mother, a CEO, or an ice cream vendor, there will always be a period in your life where you will get very busy. Especially when bills start piling up, the tendency is to work more and more. You can be as productive as you can be, but what usually happens is you forget to give attention to your one and only body. Body fat starts accumulating and body weight starts going up. You will start feeling sluggish and become easily irritated. Worse, you might start getting sick because of unhealthy eating habits and toxin build up.

You then will start being aware that you need to have a diet plan and a workout plan. But if your problem is time, how can it be possible right? If you already have financial issues, how can a gym membership still fit in your budget? Don't lose hope. As they say, if there is a will, there is a way! Well, here are some suggestions that you can choose from that will fit your lifestyle:

1. **The Scientific 8-Minute workout** – You heard it right, this workout only lasts seven minutes! It is great for people who have the busiest mornings! All you need is a mat and you're good to go! What is the Scientific 7-Minute workout about? It is actually a kind of interval training which focuses on different metabolic pathways almost at the same time. In short, it is a series of exercises that designed scientifically to work out almost every muscle group in your body. It fast. It easy to do. It is reliable. Below are the steps in the workout:
    - Jumping jacks
     -Wall sit
    -Push-up
    -Abdominal crunch
    -Step-up onto chair
    -Squat
    -Triceps dip on chair
    -Plank
    -High knees/running in place
    -Lunge
    -Push-up and rotation
    -Side plank

The goal is to do the routine 12 times, performing each exercise for 30 seconds with a 10-second rest between exercises.

2. **The Five Tibetan Rites** – This type of exercise has been around for ages. It is highly recommended for those who want to increase flexibility, are not fond of rigorous routines like the one above or those who would want to do yoga but have no time to go to classes. The Five Tibetan rites involves five poses which you would do on repetitions. Below are the descriptions for each rite:

Rite 1

Find a comfortable space and make sure it is big enough for you to wiggle a bit. Stand with your arms outstretched and horizontal to the floor with your palms facing down. Make it a point that your arms are in line with your shoulders. Then, position your feet about hip distance apart. Find a spot and focus on it while you do your rotations. The next step would be to spin around (expect to get a bit dizzy, it is okay as blood starts flowing inside your body). Little by little, increase the number of spins that you do until you are able to reach 21 spins. Feel free. Spin like a child. Remember to breathe deeply.

Rite 2

This time, you could make use of a yoga mat because you need to lie down. Then fully extend your arms along your sides and make sure that your palms are facing the floor. Inhale and raise your head off the floor. While doing so, be mindful to tuck your chin into your chest. Then, lift your legs while making sure your knees are straight and are in a vertical position. As you exhale, lower your legs to the floor while keeping your knees straight and your big toes together as long as possible. Remember to breathe deeply as you lower your legs and end your pose.

Rite 3

This time, you will need to kneel down while making sure your toes are curled under. Then you need to put your hands at the back of your thighs. After making sure that you are comfortable in your current position and that you are able to hold your ground, tuck your chin towards your chest then slide your hands down until it reaches the back of your thighs. Your shoulders should be pushed back and your head is trying to reach the sky as far as you can. Remember to arch your back and move slowly to an upright position. Repeat. Remember to exhale as you end your pose.

Rite 4

Sit down on your mat and make sure that your legs are straight and that they are in front of you. See to it that the distance between your feet are at least 12 inches apart. Look for your sitz bones (the two bony projections at the bottom of your pelvis) and place your palms alongside them. Then, gently drop your head back while you raise your torso but make sure that your knees are bent and that your arms are straight. You may rest for a few seconds before repeating the pose. Make sure that you breathe in as you rise, hold your breath for a few seconds and breath out as you release the pose.

Rite 5

You will need to lie down to do the last rite or pose. Make sure that you lie down on your belly with your palms face down. Do an upward-facing dog. Make sure to curl your toes under and lift your heart while drawing your shoulders back. Inhale and make sure that you are looking straight ahead of you. Exhale and do the downward-facing dog pose. Relax for a few seconds and repeat.

3. **The Ultimate 10-Minute workout** – What's the difference of this workout from the Scientific 7-Minute workout? This type of workout is more for those who are into the cardio stuff. The other one is more for people who wants to experience intense workouts. Here is a simple guide for those interested in the Ultimate 10-Minute workout:

The first thing to do is to do warm ups. Loosening stiff muscles are a great start for any workout or exercise routine. This is also to avoid accidents or unnecessary stretching of muscles.

- Start by circling your arms for 30 seconds

- March in place with high knees for 30 seconds

- Do 10 calf raises

- Do 10 squats

- Do 10 low lunges

- Jog in place for 30 seconds

After the warm-ups, you are now ready for the cardio exercises. Here is the list:

- EXERCISE 1: March in place like what you did in your warm-up

- EXERCISE 2: Do some shallow squats with your arms out raised front. Make sure that as you lower your body, you lift your arms in front you and that it is parallel to the floor.

- EXERCISE 3: Jog in place, be mindful of your breathing.

- EXERCISE 4: Do some slightly deeper squats while doing shoulder press at the same time. When you lower your body, fold your arms towards your chest and as you come up, do a shoulder press and then try to reach your arms as high as you can above your head.

- EXERCISE 5: Do some jumping jacks

- EXERCISE 6: Do some squats

- EXERCISE 7: Do some jumping or stepping from side to side, inhale and exhale

- EXERCISE 8: Do some split squat with shoulder shrug, do this for 30 seconds.

If time still allows, repeat the sequence. Remember to do some cooling down exercises after working out.

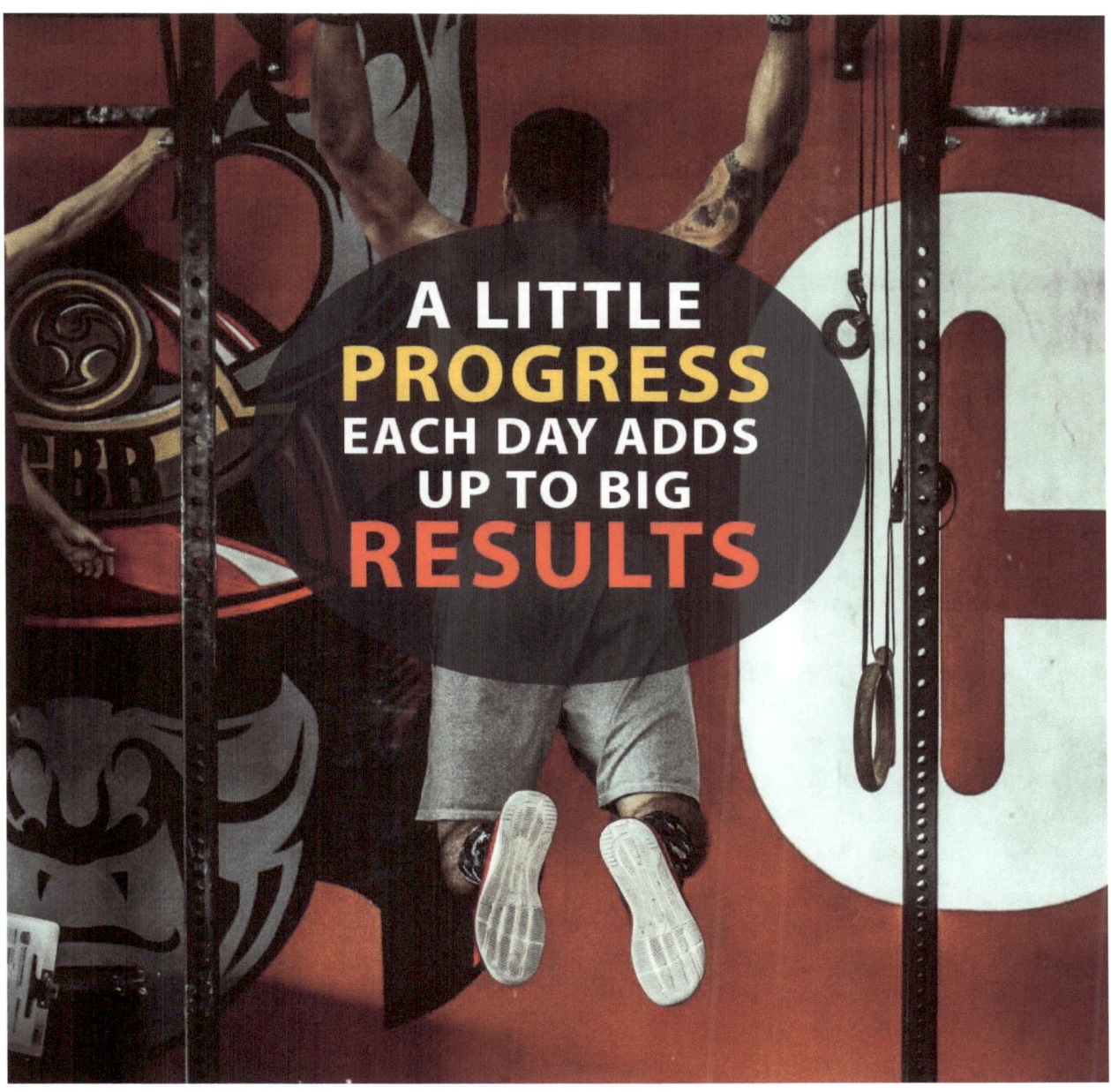

Chapter 8: Simple Yet Effective Exercises

The previous chapter presented three types of workouts you can choose from, depending on what fits your lifestyle. You can either choose a 7-Minute intense workout, a flexibility workout or a cardio workout. Although the three differs in approach, what makes it effective is the commitment you will be putting on it.

But still, if you have read and reread the previous chapter and even tried the three suggested workouts, and yet you still find yourself having a hard time choosing one or adhering to one, don't get frustrated. In any weight loss plan, there will always be challenges. Either you will have a hard time cutting down on carbs or getting to move your body. Worry not, if you have found your perfect diet plan, then finding a workout, no matter how simple, is possible and will surely aid in your weight-loss agenda. Below are simple exercises which you can choose from, depending on what suits your mornings:

Body Rolling – Roll your way to fitness if you find intense workouts too intense and you are too busy for anything more complicated than rolling. The goal of this exercise is to keep your balance, better joint alignment and blood flow. What you need is a space, first physically (you need to find a nook in your home where you can do the exercise). Then think of body rolling as also creating space for all those tight and contracted muscles which are the main reasons for not having the stamina to do exercises, body inflammation and food cravings. You will need a Yamuna ball which can be purchased online to do body rolling. Try it and check yourself if, by doing this religiously, you find yourself wanting to do more exercises, do so.

Lunges – These are great for apple-shaped body types as it strengthens the lower body where body fat tends to accumulate. It also targets flexibility and helps in the toning of the whole body. Lunges can be done anywhere, anytime. You can lunge in the kitchen while having your morning coffee, in the office while checking your emails, etc.

Planks – This exercise is ideal for those prone to accumulating body fat in their bellies. Not only is belly fat an unflattering sight, it is also kind of a stubborn kind of fat. Planks have a lot of advantages for your body. It strengthens your core muscles and this may mean healthier gut and easy digestion which you need for weight-loss.

Planks are also great for strengthening your abs and back muscles. A stronger you may mean that in time, you might be ready for more intense and fat-burning workouts. Another thing that makes planks great is that all you need to do it is a small flat surface.

Chair Dips – They say that too much seating can lower your lifespan, now don't go blaming your chair, instead, turn your "chair experience" into something positive: do some chair dips! Chair dips are low-cost, effective, strengthening exercise that is very reliable when it comes to weight-loss. The fact that you can do it anywhere and anytime makes no excuse even for the laziest health-buff wannabe. Just make sure that what you will be using is a sturdy and standard-sized chair to avoid injuries and your efforts worth all the dips.

Jump-ropes – This "tool" dates back to tale as old as time. Its simplicity – easy to carry, light weight and low-maintenance, makes it an ideal gadget for those busy people trying to lose weight. Jumping ropes are great substitutes for complicated cardio workouts and are a great calorie-burning simple exercise. The faster you jump, the greater the calories burned. What's more, jumping ropes is also great for your bone density and improving brain activity. A few tips when doing it though: for ladies, make sure that you are wearing the right kind of brassiere (as with any sport-related activity) to avoid any form of injury, for men, make sure that you have the right kind of supporter briefs to protect you. And for anyone who is interested to do this type of exercise, comfortable shoes are a plus.

Squats – Squats have been around a long time for a reason: when it comes to weight-loss or anything that involves fitness, it is an A-Lister. Mainly for reasons such as it is effective and easy to find space for. It also targets the whole body and is considered to be one of the most effective complete body exercises. It aims to target body fats and build muscle. Pairing squats with a proper diet will surely make weight-loss an easy journey instead of a frustrating and difficult one. The most important thing to remember when doing squats is proper form. Without it, efforts are just going to be wasted.

Calf raises – Calf raises are best for strengthening and toning your legs. In weight-loss, it aids in helping you build muscles instead of body fats. What's more is that you can do it at home and in your office, while caring for your child of watching your favorite T.V. show. It can also be an alternative if you are still having a difficult time doing squats. It also preps the body for more vigorous exercises. Calf raises can serve as a warm-up for bigger things as it makes your body used to moving and sweating.

Just be wary of proper form as with a lot of other exercises, proper form has a lot to do with results.

Arm circles – This is most useful, especially to women who have the tendency to accumulate fats on their arms. It is a natural mechanism of the body to store fats in the arms as it tries to protect it from injuries. But, flabby arms can also be an unsightly thing to have. As such, arm circles are an easy and easy way of making sure that toned arms are achievable. It can be done in varying intensity, duration and repetitions. Just make sure that when doing arm circles, you do proper stretches first and wait until you feel the "burn," - a signal that body fats are starting to get confused.

Jumping Jacks – A mere 100 jumping jacks done in half an hour is enough to burn around 200 calories. Isn't that amazing? In just 30 minutes, the burger and fries you have just eaten for lunch will start to get burned and won't go straight to you belly or thighs! Jumping jacks impacts flexibility and cardio. It stretches muscles and makes your heart beat faster and will also make you sweat like real pro. Aside from that, it is easy to follow (you've been doing this unconsciously since you were a child) and no tool, gadget or maintenance is required.

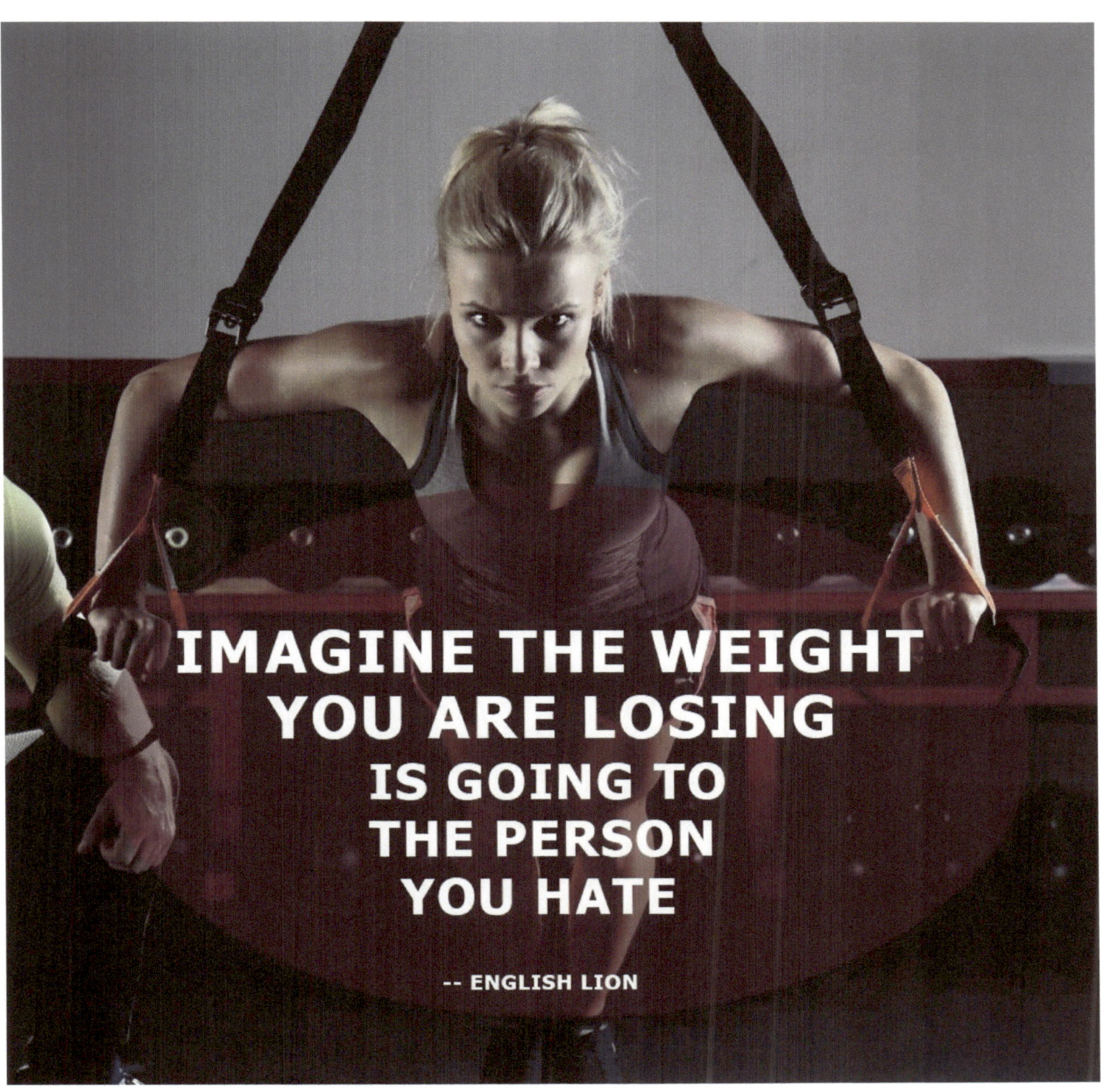

Chapter 9: Morning Light and Weight-Loss

No matter how good-sounding or what claims say, it's the most effective routine. Regardless of how passionately fitness coaches recommend a workout routine, if it won't work for you nor suit your lifestyle, it simply would just be a jumble of words and your body fats will stay where they are. So how does one find a weight-loss routine that matters? And what if you are too busy to look for what suits you? Well, let's get realistic here and appreciate the fact that you have already acknowledged that you need to lose weight. However, if you still haven't got the right timing yet to do everything you've been planning, here are tips that may serve as "transition" activities so as not to waste your initial efforts.

Make sure to start your mornings right. This is because, the truth is, how you start your day has a lot to do with losing weight. Remember that mornings signal a new day, a new beginning and another chance to set things right!

Make sure to begin you day with a lot of sunshine or vitamin D. This is because basking in the sun not only is good for your physical health but to your emotional health as well. In a study conducted by fitness experts, they concluded that those who are able to get vitamin D in the mornings have higher metabolisms and as a result, have lower cravings for unhealthy food during the rest of their day. On the other hand, people who prefer to spend their mornings in the dark tend to have slower metabolisms and as a result, crave for sugar and carbs during the day. Morning light has a natural effect on one's circadian rhythm or biological clock. This means that it has an effect on your internal clock, sleeping habits and immune system – all these are crucial to weight-loss. What's more is that sunlight is free, all you need to do is to get out of your room for 30 to 40 minutes in the morning or late afternoon and that's it.

Make sure that you are sleeping well and enough. This means that your sleep should be uninterrupted and that you don't need the constant rings of an alarm clock to wake you up. Keep in mind that your sleep patterns greatly affect your weight. It may sound cliché but it is a hard truth. How well you have rested through the night will dictate your cravings for the day. Lack of sleep causes the body to crave sugar in order to make up for lost energy.

Aside from that, lack of proper sleep makes you not so good in decision-making when it comes to whether you are to order a salad bowl or a large fries for brunch. An average of 8 hours is ideal to say that you have rested well for the night.

Make mindfulness a goal the moment you open your eyes. This is because this state of mind is an important key factor in weight loss. How so? Mindfulness means taking control of your thoughts. If you believe in your goals and remind yourself of it the moment you wake up, you set your thinking that whatever it is that you have set as your goal can be made a reality. It keeps you focused throughout your day and makes you say no to binge-eating and other actions that go against your weight-loss goals. When you are mindful, you will remember to do your morning exercise, you will also more likely choose a healthier alternative for breakfast and the rest of your meals for the day. To help yourself be mindful, take deep breaths as you wake up and focus on even breaths. Play in your mind your agenda for the day and if you can, mentally picture your meals and exercise routine, no matter how simple. Be happy about it and try to stay positive.

Encourage yourself. Alter the way you commute to work or to your kid's school. There are a lot of ways you can squeeze exercise to the simple task of getting to where you are supposed to be for the day. Depending on your geographical location, biking, walking, jogging can be healthy alternatives to riding. If stairs do get involved, the better. What's important is that you are able to get your body moving even if it is just for a matter of a few minutes. At the end of each week or month, try making a journal of the little miles where you chose walking over car rides and you will be surprised to know that when they all add up, it can be equal to hours spent in a gym. The perk of it is that, you didn't get to spend money for classes and that it was subconsciously done. Make it an effort to try this until it becomes a habit of yours.

Get to know protein more. Why protein? This is because when trying to lose weight, a healthy dose pf protein starting from your breakfast will make you lose pounds of belly fat. To eat breakfast like a king is one of the truths a person trying to lose weight needs to believe in. Skipping this important meal can create havoc throughout your day. If you are so busy and our mornings already lack time, try the scheme of preparing your breakfast before you go to sleep (think overnight oats). For those having a hard time eating full meals in the mornings, chia pudding (recipes are abundant in the internet) and green smoothies spiked with superfood is a great way to start. Here is a list of protein-packed food that you may want to start including not only in your breakfast but in your diet as well:

- broccoli
- Greek yogurt
- rolled oats

43

- almonds
- chicken breasts
- eggs
- cottage cheese
- whole wheat bread
- lentils
- quinoa
- lean beef
- tuna

Make it a habit to pack your snacks if you really are serious about your weight loss goal. Admittedly, it is easier to buy a doughnut than look for a fat-free, low-carb snack in your canteen. And you can't help but buy that sugar-laden doughnut if you are too busy, right? The solution? Pack your snacks like what your mother did when you were in elementary! This way, you will still be able to control your calorie intake and refrain yourself from eating what is readily available around you that is most of the time unhealthy. Here is a list of sample healthy snacks that you can pack:

- dark chocolate
- nuts
- unsalted butter-free popcorn
- grapes
- chickpeas
- cherry tomatoes with blue cheese toppings
- celery sticks stuffed with peanut butter
- cucumber with hummus for dipping
- kale chips
- hard-boiled eggs
- carrot sticks

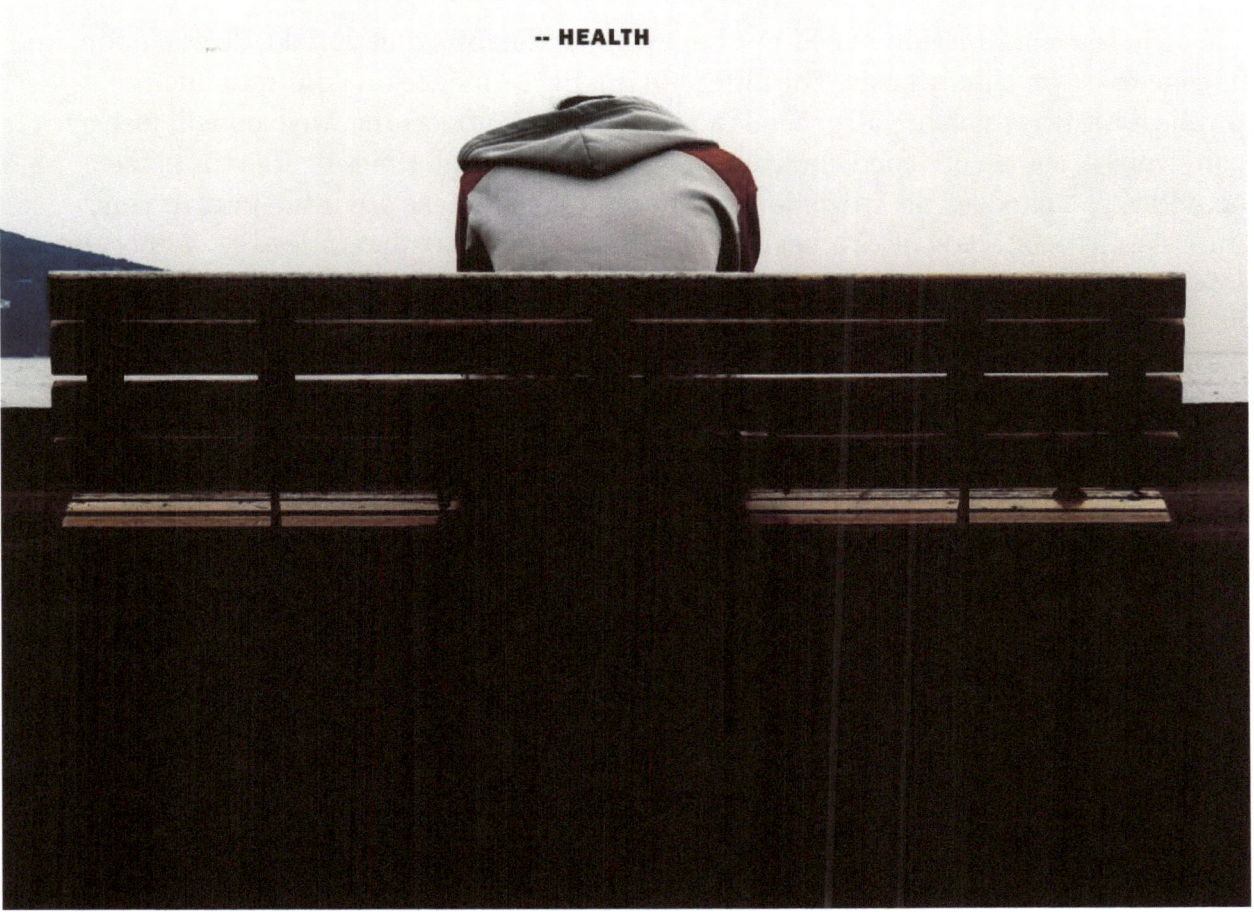

Chapter 10: Lifestyle, Brain Rewiring and Weight-Loss

In the previous chapters of this book, you've been advised that the test to any workout routine is to notice if it mentions a lifestyle change. If it is never mentioned, then red flag is up – it usually is a fad or a hype. The truth is that, no matter how busy you are, without a change in lifestyle, weight-loss and even maintaining weight-loss is next to impossible.

Lifestyle is a combination of actions, behaviors and habits that you do, decide upon, and engage to do on a daily basis. Your lifestyle is a big influence on your mental and physical health which are all crucial in weight-loss. It affects the way you will lose or gain weight, a lot. Your food choices, how you spend break times or free time, the activities you choose add movement to your body – all these are influences to your lifestyle. If you already have a healthy diet, then we can say that indeed, you may already lose weight. But in order to maintain it, you need to make an effort to incorporate more healthy habits to your lifestyle. Here is a list of what we can consider as simple healthy habits that aid in weight-loss, especially for busy people:

- Plan your meals ahead of time

- Eat slowly and chew your food well (putting your fork down between bites)

- Drink lots of water

- Don't skip breakfast

- Always have a simple snack with you (apple, banana or carrot)

- Exercise even when you don't feel like it

- Accept your body type. The key is to know where your fats get stored and target it on your next exercise routine.

- Know when you are really hungry, know when you are emotionally hungry

- Practice rationing your portions and be disciplined about it

- Choose fruits as desserts

Keep in mind that in order to achieve a healthier lifestyle, a series of changes in diet, behavior and thinking patterns are needed. Reverting back to unhealthy habits is usually the reason why when one has already achieved his ideal weight, keeping it does not take place. It takes more than an instant diet to keep your body healthy for a long time or better, a lifetime. Keep in mind that what we sometimes refer to as small behaviors make a great impact in our overall health. To make things clearer, here are examples of seemingly small behaviors that are actually unhealthy:

1. Not drinking enough water
2. Poor sleeping habits
3. Not minding stress levels
4. Making excuses for not exercising
5. Relying on to-go food
6. Not being mindful of how you spend your free time

The list above is are just samples of small behaviors that greatly affect your health. The list could go on but leaning on the positive side, the first thing to do if you really want to lose weight despite your busy schedule is to recognize your current habits, know what needs changing and start developing healthier habits – ones that you can live with for the rest of your life.

How to Develop Healthy Habits?

Know that it takes at least 66 days to develop a new habit. You heard that right. For someone to be able to have a new solid habit, it needs to be practiced for at least two months. This means that you need to have patience if you want to develop something. Be it a new habit in eating or exercising, you may need to wait until it enters your whole being and becomes a part of you. So, don't get easily frustrated if you experience setbacks or failures at first. Try to keep your motivation and always keep your goal as your inspiration.

Take time to study how a habit works, its roots and where it is coming from before trying to change it. A habit can be broken down into three actions: a cue, which is the trigger that makes you do the habit; a routine, which is essentially the action you do automatically; and the rewards, which is the rewarding feeling you get after doing the action. To further understand, let's take a look at this example – when trying to exercise in the morning, you need to have your cue – it may be the sight of your yoga mat or your favorite jam on Spotify. Then routine comes next. Since this is automatic, your body will already know what to do, it has in its muscle memory the sequence of the exercise routine that you are to do. Lastly, the reward. This may be the digits that you see in your weighing scale. It is what keeps you motivated and excited to do the habit all over again the next day. Now that you know how a habit works, you can decide how to make a healthy practice into a habit.

Keep in mind that variety is not your friend when trying to establish a habit. This is because habit creation means repeating a single action until it is deeply embedded in your memory and muscle memory. This means to say eating the same banana with our oats every single day at breakfast. When you try to add an apple in day 5 and then decide to change it to grapefruit in day 12, then your goal of creating a habit is tinged with a bit of confusion. Just keep in mind that you need to stick to the same routine every single day until it has become a habit. Choosing to have variations extends the amount of time it takes to reach goal and your motivation comes with a lot more effort.

If in case you miss a day, don't lose hope. Remember that you are but human and bound to make mistakes. What's important is that you stick to your goals until you have reach them. Remember that attitude, when it comes to habit forming, is as important as sticking to it.

Now that you have reach the final chapter of this book, it is time to act upon your weight loss goals.

10 WEIGHT LOSS
SECRETS FOR BUSY PEOPLE

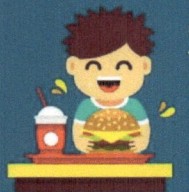

ONLY EAT WHEN YOU'RE HUNGRY
Not because you are bored miserable or because you must try that new Tim Tam Flavor (and then devour the packet)

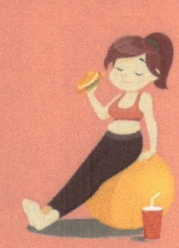

EAT LESS
Sorry, no way to avoid that one. Eat smaller portions. Eat dinner on entree sized plates and when eating out, always order an entree for main

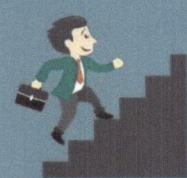

MOVE MORE
Take advantage of incidental exercise. Take the stairs or walk to the shops instead of taking the car

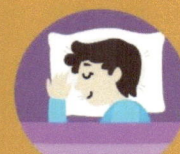

GET ENOUGH SLEEP
Tired people have increased ghrelin, a harmone which stimulates appetite.

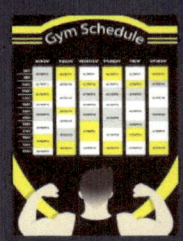

PLAN IN EXERCISE
Schedule it into your diary or phone just like an appointment and treat it like one

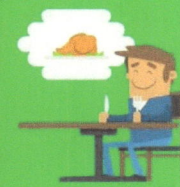

YOUR FAVORITE FOODS
Didn't we just tell you to not eat any more Tim Tams? If you want a treat, make it yourself and make it healthy.

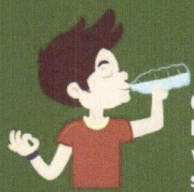

DRINK WATER OFTEN
6-8 glasses a day is ideal Hunger is often confused with thirst and dehydration so drink before you eat

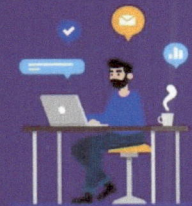

FOCUS ON WHAT'S MOTIVATING YOU
A note, a photo or a quote, keep it with you for a constant reminder of why you want to change.

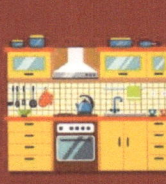

GET ORGANIZED IN THE KITCHEN
Create a healthy meal plan for the week, write a shopping lis (and stick to it) Prepare meals and snack in advance. A little planning means you avoid the 5pm dinner panic

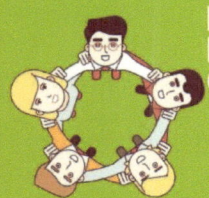

FINALLY EMBRACE CHANGE
Because you can't expect to do the same thing over and over and suddenly get different results!

Checklists

CHECKLIST 1

How To Keep Yourself From Getting Frustrated In Your Weight Loss Journey

- Accept that there is no alternative to exercising regularly

- Before getting frustrated, make sure that you have no medical condition that makes you gain weight no matter what you do

- Believe that there is a strong connection between sleep and weight gain

- Make water you best friend

CHECKLIST 2

How To Spot A Fad Diet Product

1. Weight loss is based on taking pills, powders, special juices or herbs

2. Weight loss is based on drastically cutting back on calories

3. Weight loss is based on skipping meals and replacing them with special shakes/drinks or food bars

4. Weight loss plans that promises instant results

5. Weight loss plans that never mentions lifestyle or change in mentality

CHECKLIST 3

How To Start Your Day Towards Positive Weight Loss

- Make sure to begin you day with a lot of sunshine or vitamin D

- Make sure that you are sleeping well and enough

- Make mindfulness a goal the moment you open your eyes

- Alter the way you commute to work or to your kid's school

- Get to know protein more

- Make it a habit to pack your snacks if you really are serious about your weight loss goal

CHECKLIST 4

Healthier Options for On-The-Go Snacks

1. Dark chocolate
2. Nuts
3. Unsalted butter-free popcorn
4. Grapes
5. Chickpeas
6. Cherry tomatoes with blue cheese toppings
7. Celery sticks (optional: cream cheese dipping)
8. Cucumber (optional: hummus dipping)
9. Kale chips
10. Hard-boiled eggs
11. Carrot sticks

CHECKLIST 5

Simple Healthy Habits That Aid In Weight-Loss For Busy People
- Plan your meals ahead of time

- Eat slowly and chew your food well

- Drink lots of water

- Don't skip breakfast

- Always have a simple snack with you (apple, banana or carrot)

- Exercise even when you don't feel like it

- Accept your body type. The key is to know where your fats get stored and target it on your next exercise routine.

- Know when you are really hungry, know when you are emotionally hungry

- Practice rationing your portions and be disciplined about it

- Choose fruits as desserts

About the Author

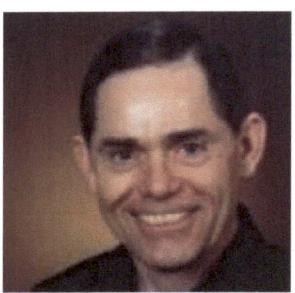

I have published numerous books on Amazon for Kindle and other publishing platforms. Both in electronic and POD formats.

While most of my books are on health and fitness in general, my topics of interest are leaning more toward aging baby boomers and the older population.

Besides my own writing, I also ghostwrite ebooks, books, reports, articles, blogs and do Kindle conversions for clients on a variety of topics. Go to my website at http://ronknesswriting.com for more information or to submit a quote. For a complete list of my books, go to https://www.amazon.com/Ron-Kness/e/B0072M6PYO.

Today my wife and I are retired from our careers and live in San Tan Valley, AZ. I now write as a retirement business where you'll find me happily sitting in my office typing away on my laptop as I work on my next book or ghostwriting project . . . that is if we are not traveling on a cruise ship - our new-found mode of travel.